THIS BOOK BELONGS TO

NAME:

_____

ADDRESS:

_____

_____

_____

Phone Number:

_____

Favorite Scripture:

_____

_____

_____

_____

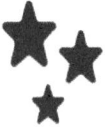

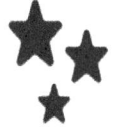

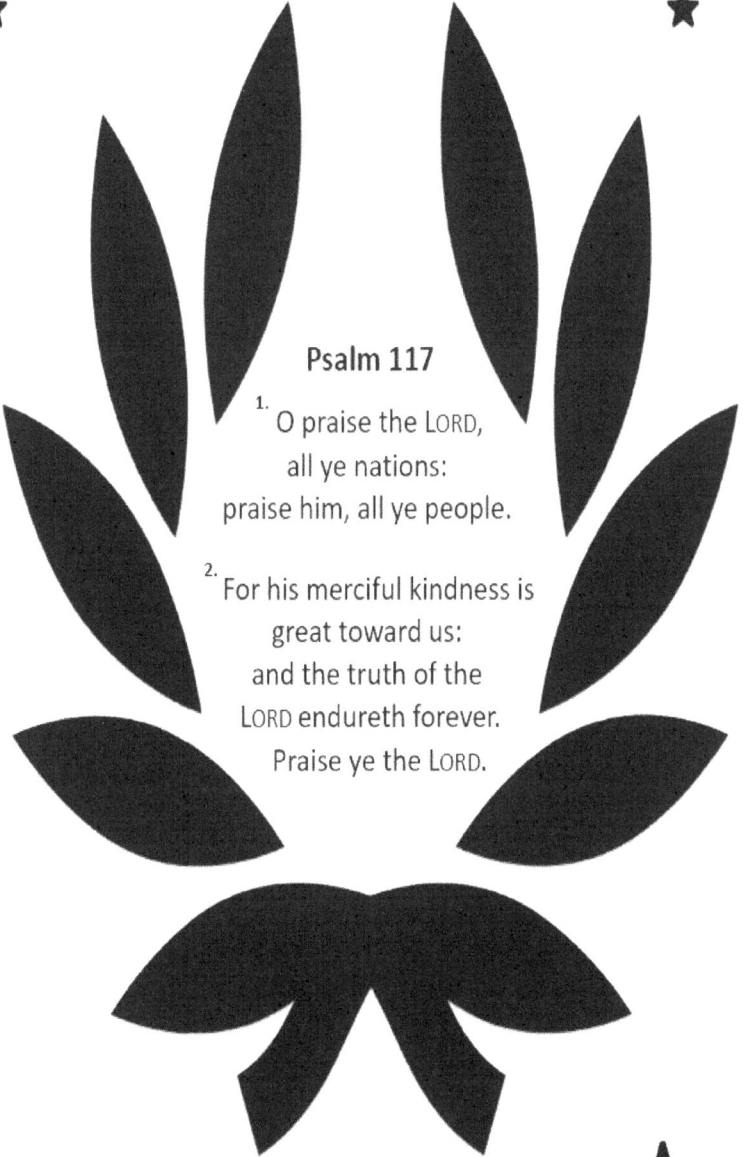

Psalm 117

1. O praise the LORD,
all ye nations:
praise him, all ye people.

2. For his merciful kindness is
great toward us:
and the truth of the
LORD endureth forever.
Praise ye the LORD.

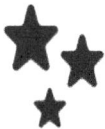

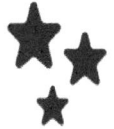

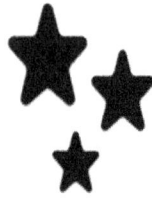

Psalm 18:3

I will call upon the LORD,
who is worthy to be praised:
so shall I be saved from my
enemies.

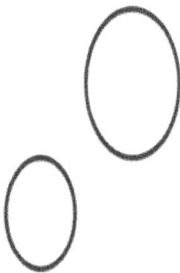

Date:

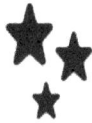

Verse of The Day: _____
_____
_____
_____

Prayer Requests:

Praise Reports:

Reflections: _____
_____
_____
_____
_____

Date:

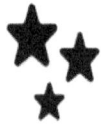

Verse of The Day: _____
_____
_____
_____

Prayer Requests:

Praise Reports:

Reflections: _____
_____
_____
_____
_____

Date:

Verse of The Day: _____
_____
_____
_____

Prayer Requests:

Praise Reports:

Reflections: _____
_____
_____
_____
_____

Date:

Verse of The Day: _____
_____
_____
_____

Prayer Requests:

Praise Reports:

Reflections: _____
_____
_____
_____
_____

Date:

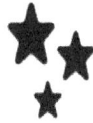

Verse of The Day:
_____
_____
_____
_____

Prayer Requests:

Praise Reports:

Reflections:
_____
_____
_____
_____
_____

Date:

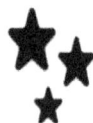

Verse of The Day: _____
_____
_____
_____

Prayer Requests:

Praise Reports:

Reflections: _____
_____
_____
_____
_____

Date:

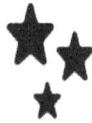

Verse of The Day: _____
_____
_____
_____

Prayer Requests:

Praise Reports:

Reflections: _____
_____
_____
_____
_____

Date:

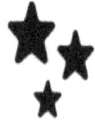

Verse of The Day: _____
_____
_____
_____

Prayer Requests:

Praise Reports:

Reflections: _____
_____
_____
_____
_____

Date:

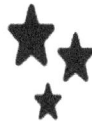

Verse of The Day: _____
_____
_____
_____

Prayer Requests:

Praise Reports:

Reflections: _____
_____
_____
_____
_____

Date:

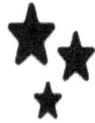

Verse of The Day: _____
_____
_____
_____

Prayer Requests:

Praise Reports:

Reflections: _____
_____
_____
_____
_____

Date:

Verse of The Day: _____
_____
_____
_____

Prayer Requests:

Praise Reports:

Reflections: _____
_____
_____
_____
_____

Date: _____

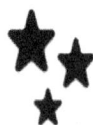

Verse of The Day: _____
_____
_____
_____

Prayer Requests:

Praise Reports:

Reflections: _____
_____
_____
_____
_____

Date:

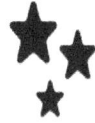

Verse of The Day: _____
_____
_____
_____

Prayer Requests:

Praise Reports:

Reflections: _____
_____
_____
_____
_____

Date:

Verse of The Day: _____
_____
_____
_____

Prayer Requests:

Praise Reports:

Reflections: _____
_____
_____
_____
_____

Date:

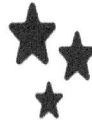

Verse of The Day: _____
_____
_____
_____

Prayer Requests:

Praise Reports:

Reflections: _____
_____
_____
_____
_____

Date:

Verse of The Day: _____
_____
_____
_____

Prayer Requests:

Praise Reports:

Reflections:_____
_____
_____
_____
_____

Date: ★ ★ ★

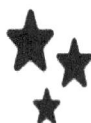

Verse of The Day: _____
_____
_____
_____

Prayer Requests:

Praise Reports:

Reflections: _____
_____
_____
_____
_____

Date:

Verse of The Day: _____
_____
_____
_____

Prayer Requests:

Praise Reports:

Reflections: _____
_____
_____
_____
_____

Date:

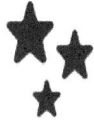

Verse of The Day: _____
_____
_____
_____

Prayer Requests:

Praise Reports:

Reflections: _____
_____
_____
_____
_____

Date:

Verse of The Day: _____
_____
_____
_____

Prayer Requests:

Praise Reports:

Reflections: _____
_____
_____
_____
_____

Date:

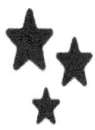

Verse of The Day: _____
_____
_____
_____

Prayer Requests:

Praise Reports:

Reflections: _____
_____
_____
_____
_____

Date:

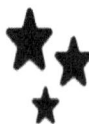

Verse of The Day: _____
_____
_____
_____

Prayer Requests:

Praise Reports:

Reflections: _____
_____
_____
_____
_____

Date:

Verse of The Day: _____
_____
_____
_____

Prayer Requests:

Praise Reports:

Reflections: _____
_____
_____
_____
_____

Date:

Verse of The Day: _____
_____
_____
_____

Prayer Requests:

Praise Reports:

Reflections: _____
_____
_____
_____
_____

Date:

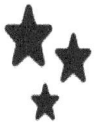

Verse of The Day: _____
_____
_____
_____

Prayer Requests:

Praise Reports:

Reflections: _____
_____
_____
_____
_____

Date:

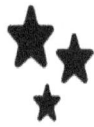

Verse of The Day: _____
_____
_____
_____

Prayer Requests:

Praise Reports:

Reflections: _____
_____
_____
_____
_____

Date:

Verse of The Day: _____
_____
_____
_____
_____

Prayer Requests:

Praise Reports:

Reflections: _____
_____
_____
_____
_____

Date:

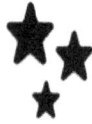

Verse of The Day: _____
_____
_____
_____

Prayer Requests:

Praise Reports:

Reflections: _____
_____
_____
_____
_____

Date:

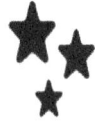

Verse of The Day: _____
_____
_____
_____

Prayer Requests:

Praise Reports:

Reflections: _____
_____
_____
_____
_____

Date:

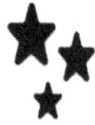

Verse of The Day: _____
_____
_____
_____

Prayer Requests:

Praise Reports:

Reflections: _____
_____
_____
_____
_____

Date:

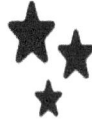

Verse of The Day: _____
_____
_____
_____

Prayer Requests:

Praise Reports:

Reflections: _____
_____
_____
_____
_____

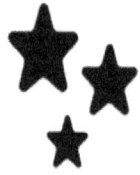

Nehemiah 8:10
The joy of the Lord is my
strength.

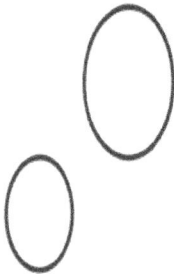

Date:

Verse of The Day: _____
_____
_____
_____
_____

Prayer Requests:

Praise Reports:

Reflections: _____
_____
_____
_____
_____
_____

Date:

Verse of The Day: _____
_____
_____
_____
_____

Prayer Requests:

Praise Reports:

Reflections: _____
_____
_____
_____
_____

Date:

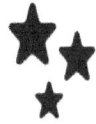

Verse of The Day: _____
_____
_____
_____
_____

Prayer Requests:

Praise Reports:

Reflections: _____
_____
_____
_____
_____
_____

Date:

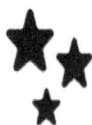

Verse of The Day: _____
_____
_____
_____

Prayer Requests:

Praise Reports:

Reflections: _____
_____
_____
_____
_____

Date:

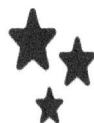

Verse of The Day: _____
_____
_____
_____
_____

Prayer Requests:

Praise Reports:

Reflections: _____
_____
_____
_____
_____

Date:

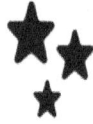

Verse of The Day: _____
_____
_____
_____

Prayer Requests:

Praise Reports:

Reflections: _____
_____
_____
_____
_____

Date:

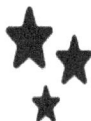

Verse of The Day: _____
_____
_____
_____

Prayer Requests:

Praise Reports:

Reflections: _____
_____
_____
_____
_____

Date:

Verse of The Day: _____
_____
_____
_____

Prayer Requests:

Praise Reports:

Reflections: _____
_____
_____
_____
_____

Date:

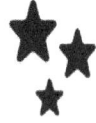

Verse of The Day: _____
_____
_____
_____

Prayer Requests:

Praise Reports:

Reflections: _____
_____
_____
_____
_____

Date:

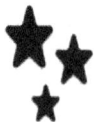

Verse of The Day: _____
_____
_____
_____

Prayer Requests:

Praise Reports:

Reflections: _____
_____
_____
_____
_____

Date:

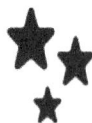

Verse of The Day: _____
_____
_____
_____
_____

Prayer Requests:

Praise Reports:

Reflections: _____
_____
_____
_____
_____

Date:

Verse of The Day: _____
_____
_____
_____

Prayer Requests:

Praise Reports:

Reflections: _____
_____
_____
_____
_____

Date:

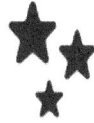

Verse of The Day: _____
_____
_____
_____

Prayer Requests:

Praise Reports:

Reflections: _____
_____
_____
_____
_____

Date:

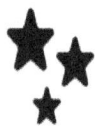

Verse of The Day: _____
_____
_____
_____

Prayer Requests:

Praise Reports:

Reflections: _____
_____
_____
_____
_____

Date:

Verse of The Day: _____
_____
_____
_____

Prayer Requests:

Praise Reports:

Reflections: _____
_____
_____
_____
_____

Date:

Verse of The Day: _____
_____
_____
_____

Prayer Requests:

Praise Reports:

Reflections: _____
_____
_____
_____
_____

Date:

Verse of The Day: _____
_____
_____
_____

Prayer Requests:

Praise Reports:

Reflections: _____
_____
_____
_____
_____

Date:

Verse of The Day: _____
_____
_____
_____

Prayer Requests:

Praise Reports:

Reflections: _____
_____
_____
_____
_____

Date:

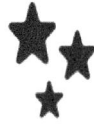

Verse of The Day: _____
_____
_____
_____

Prayer Requests:

Praise Reports:

Reflections: _____
_____
_____
_____
_____

Date:

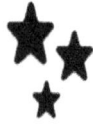

Verse of The Day: _____
_____
_____
_____
_____

Prayer Requests:

Praise Reports:

Reflections: _____
_____
_____
_____
_____

Date:

Verse of The Day: _____
_____
_____
_____

Prayer Requests:

Praise Reports:

Reflections: _____
_____
_____
_____
_____

Date:

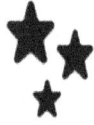

Verse of The Day: _____
_____
_____
_____

Prayer Requests:

Praise Reports:

Reflections: _____
_____
_____
_____
_____

Date:

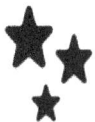

Verse of The Day:

_____
_____
_____
_____
_____

Prayer Requests:

Praise Reports:

Reflections:

_____
_____
_____
_____
_____

Date:

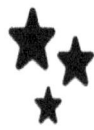

Verse of The Day: _____
_____
_____
_____
_____

Prayer Requests:

Praise Reports:

Reflections: _____
_____
_____
_____
_____

Date:

Verse of The Day: _____
_____
_____
_____

Prayer Requests:

Praise Reports:

Reflections: _____
_____
_____
_____
_____

Date:

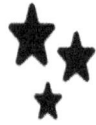

Verse of The Day: _____
_____
_____
_____

Prayer Requests:

Praise Reports:

Reflections: _____
_____
_____
_____
_____

Date:

Verse of The Day: _____
_____
_____
_____

Prayer Requests:

Praise Reports:

Reflections: _____
_____
_____
_____
_____

Date:

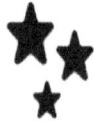

Verse of The Day: _____
_____
_____
_____

Prayer Requests:

Praise Reports:

Reflections: _____
_____
_____
_____
_____

Date:

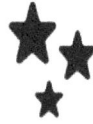

Verse of The Day: _____
_____
_____
_____

Prayer Requests:

Praise Reports:

Reflections: _____
_____
_____
_____
_____

Date:

Verse of The Day: _____
_____
_____
_____

Prayer Requests:

Praise Reports:

Reflections: _____
_____
_____
_____
_____

Date:

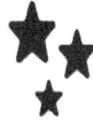

Verse of The Day: _____
_____
_____
_____

Prayer Requests:

Praise Reports:

Reflections: _____
_____
_____
_____
_____

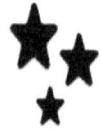

2 Corinthians 5:7

For I walk by faith,
not by sight

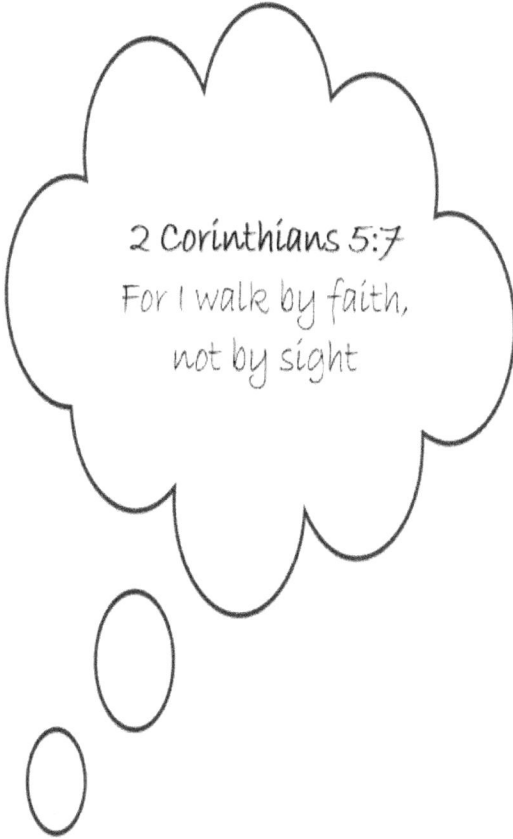

Date:

Verse of The Day: _____

_____

_____

_____

Prayer Requests:

Praise Reports:

Reflections: _____

_____

_____

_____

Date:

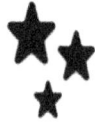

Verse of The Day: _____
_____
_____
_____

Prayer Requests:

Praise Reports:

Reflections: _____
_____
_____
_____
_____

Date:

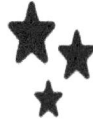

Verse of The Day: _____
_____
_____
_____

Prayer Requests:

Praise Reports:

Reflections: _____
_____
_____
_____
_____

Date:

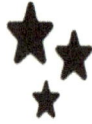

Verse of The Day: _____
_____
_____
_____

Prayer Requests:

Praise Reports:

Reflections: _____
_____
_____
_____
_____

Date:

Verse of The Day: _____
_____
_____
_____

Prayer Requests:

Praise Reports:

Reflections: _____
_____
_____
_____
_____

Date:

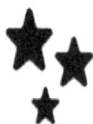

Verse of The Day: _____
_____
_____
_____

Prayer Requests:

Praise Reports:

Reflections: _____
_____
_____
_____
_____

Date:

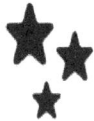

Verse of The Day: _____
_____
_____
_____

Prayer Requests:

Praise Reports:

Reflections: _____
_____
_____
_____
_____

Date:

Verse of The Day: _____
_____
_____
_____

Prayer Requests:

Praise Reports:

Reflections: _____
_____
_____
_____
_____

Date:

Verse of The Day: _____
_____
_____
_____

Prayer Requests:

Praise Reports:

Reflections: _____
_____
_____
_____
_____

Date:

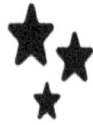

Verse of The Day: _____
_____
_____
_____

Prayer Requests:

Praise Reports:

Reflections: _____
_____
_____
_____
_____

Date:

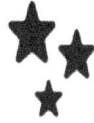

Verse of The Day: _____
_____
_____
_____

Prayer Requests:

Praise Reports:

Reflections: _____
_____
_____
_____
_____

Date:

Verse of The Day: _____
_____
_____
_____
_____

Prayer Requests:

Praise Reports:

Reflections: _____
_____
_____
_____
_____

Date:

Verse of The Day: _____
_____
_____
_____

Prayer Requests:

Praise Reports:

Reflections: _____
_____
_____
_____
_____

Date:

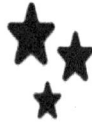

Verse of The Day: _____
_____
_____
_____

Prayer Requests:

Praise Reports:

Reflections: _____
_____
_____
_____
_____

Date:

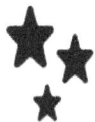

Verse of The Day: _____
_____
_____
_____

Prayer Requests:

Praise Reports:

Reflections: _____
_____
_____
_____
_____

Date:

Verse of The Day: _____
_____
_____
_____

Prayer Requests:

Praise Reports:

Reflections: _____
_____
_____
_____
_____

Date:

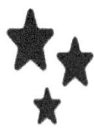

Verse of The Day: _____
_____
_____
_____

Prayer Requests:

Praise Reports:

Reflections: _____
_____
_____
_____
_____

Date:

Verse of The Day: _____
_____
_____
_____

Prayer Requests:

Praise Reports:

Reflections: _____
_____
_____
_____
_____

Date:

Verse of The Day: _____
_____
_____
_____
_____

Prayer Requests:

Praise Reports:

Reflections: _____
_____
_____
_____
_____

Date:

Verse of The Day: _____
_____
_____
_____

Prayer Requests:

Praise Reports:

Reflections: _____
_____
_____
_____
_____

Date:

Verse of The Day: _____
_____
_____
_____

Prayer Requests:

Praise Reports:

Reflections: _____
_____
_____
_____
_____

Date:

Verse of The Day: _____
_____
_____
_____

Prayer Requests:

Praise Reports:

Reflections: _____
_____
_____
_____
_____

Date:

Verse of The Day: _____
_____
_____
_____
_____

Prayer Requests:

Praise Reports:

Reflections: _____
_____
_____
_____
_____

Date:

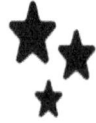

Verse of The Day: _____
_____
_____
_____

Prayer Requests:

Praise Reports:

Reflections: _____
_____
_____
_____
_____

Date:

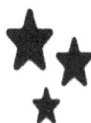

Verse of The Day: _____
_____
_____
_____

Prayer Requests:

Praise Reports:

Reflections: _____
_____
_____
_____
_____
_____

Date:

Verse of The Day: _____
_____
_____
_____

Prayer Requests:

Praise Reports:

Reflections: _____
_____
_____
_____
_____

Date:

Verse of The Day: _____
_____
_____
_____

Prayer Requests:

Praise Reports:

Reflections: _____
_____
_____
_____
_____

Date:

Verse of The Day:
_____
_____
_____
_____

Prayer Requests:

Praise Reports:

Reflections:
_____
_____
_____
_____
_____

Date:

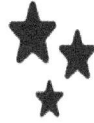

Verse of The Day: _____
_____
_____
_____

Prayer Requests:

Praise Reports:

Reflections: _____
_____
_____
_____
_____

Date:

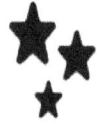

Verse of The Day: _____
_____
_____
_____

Prayer Requests:

Praise Reports:

Reflections: _____
_____
_____
_____
_____

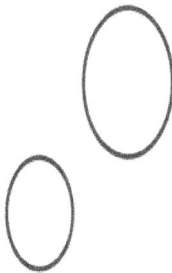

Psalm 46:1-2
God is my refuge and
strength,
an ever present help in
trouble;
Therefore, I will not
fear.

Date:

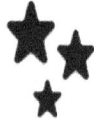

Verse of The Day: _____
_____
_____
_____
_____

Prayer Requests:

Praise Reports:

Reflections: _____
_____
_____
_____
_____

Date:

Verse of The Day: _____
_____
_____
_____

Prayer Requests:

Praise Reports:

Reflections: _____
_____
_____
_____
_____

Date:

Verse of The Day: _____
_____
_____
_____

Prayer Requests:

Praise Reports:

Reflections: _____
_____
_____
_____
_____

Date:

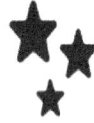

Verse of The Day: _____
_____
_____
_____
_____

Prayer Requests:

Praise Reports:

Reflections: _____
_____
_____
_____
_____

Date:

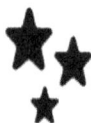

Verse of The Day: _____
_____
_____
_____

Prayer Requests:

Praise Reports:

Reflections: _____
_____
_____
_____
_____

Date:

Verse of The Day: _____
_____
_____
_____

Prayer Requests:

Praise Reports:

Reflections: _____
_____
_____
_____
_____

Date:

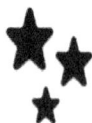

Verse of The Day: _____
_____
_____
_____

Prayer Requests:

Praise Reports:

Reflections: _____
_____
_____
_____
_____

Date:

Verse of The Day: _____
_____
_____
_____

Prayer Requests:

Praise Reports:

Reflections: _____
_____
_____
_____
_____

Date:

Verse of The Day: _____
_____
_____
_____

Prayer Requests:

Praise Reports:

Reflections:_____
_____
_____
_____
_____

Date:

Verse of The Day: _____
_____
_____
_____

Prayer Requests:

Praise Reports:

Reflections: _____
_____
_____
_____
_____

Date:

Verse of The Day: _____
_____
_____
_____

Prayer Requests:

Praise Reports:

Reflections: _____
_____
_____
_____
_____

Date:

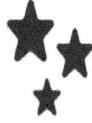

Verse of The Day: _____

_____

_____

_____

Prayer Requests:

Praise Reports:

Reflections: _____

_____

_____

_____

_____

Date:

Verse of The Day: _____
_____
_____
_____

Prayer Requests:

Praise Reports:

Reflections: _____
_____
_____
_____
_____

Date:

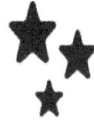

Verse of The Day: _____
_____
_____
_____

Prayer Requests:

Praise Reports:

Reflections: _____
_____
_____
_____
_____

Date:

Verse of The Day: _____
_____
_____
_____
_____

Prayer Requests:

Praise Reports:

Reflections: _____
_____
_____
_____
_____

Date:

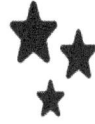

Verse of The Day: _____
_____
_____
_____
_____

Prayer Requests:

Praise Reports:

Reflections: _____
_____
_____
_____
_____

Date:

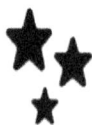

Verse of The Day: _____
_____
_____
_____

Prayer Requests:

Praise Reports:

Reflections: _____
_____
_____
_____
_____

Date:

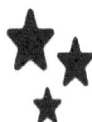

Verse of The Day: _____
_____
_____
_____

Prayer Requests:

Praise Reports:

Reflections: _____
_____
_____
_____
_____

Date:

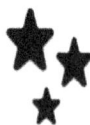

Verse of The Day: _____
_____
_____
_____

Prayer Requests:

Praise Reports:

Reflections: _____
_____
_____
_____
_____

Date:

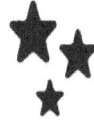

Verse of The Day: _____
_____
_____
_____

Prayer Requests:

Praise Reports:

Reflections: _____
_____
_____
_____
_____

Date:

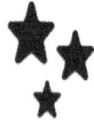

Verse of The Day: _____
_____
_____
_____
_____

Prayer Requests:

Praise Reports:

Reflections: _____
_____
_____
_____
_____

Date:

Verse of The Day: _____
_____
_____
_____
_____

Prayer Requests:

Praise Reports:

Reflections: _____
_____
_____
_____
_____

Date: _____

Verse of The Day: _____
_____
_____
_____
_____

Prayer Requests:

Praise Reports:

Reflections: _____
_____
_____
_____
_____

Date:

Verse of The Day: _____
_____
_____
_____

Prayer Requests:

Praise Reports:

Reflections: _____
_____
_____
_____
_____

Date:

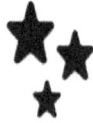

Verse of The Day: _____
_____
_____
_____

Prayer Requests:

Praise Reports:

Reflections: _____
_____
_____
_____
_____

Date:

Verse of The Day: _____
_____
_____
_____

Prayer Requests:

Praise Reports:

Reflections: _____
_____
_____
_____
_____

Date:

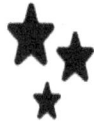

Verse of The Day: _____
_____
_____
_____

Prayer Requests:

Praise Reports:

Reflections: _____
_____
_____
_____
_____

Date:

Verse of The Day: _____
_____
_____
_____

Prayer Requests:

Praise Reports:

Reflections: _____
_____
_____
_____
_____

Date:

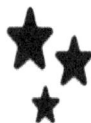

Verse of The Day: _____
_____
_____
_____

Prayer Requests:

Praise Reports:

Reflections: _____
_____
_____
_____
_____

Date:

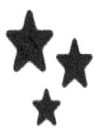

Verse of The Day: _____
_____
_____
_____

Prayer Requests:

Praise Reports:

Reflections: _____
_____
_____
_____
_____

Date:

Verse of The Day: _____
_____
_____
_____

Prayer Requests:

Praise Reports:

Reflections: _____
_____
_____
_____
_____

Psalm 5:1-2

Give ear to my words,
O Lord, consider my
meditation.
Hearken unto the voice of
my cry, my king, and
my God:
For unto thee, will I pray.

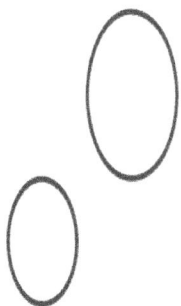

Date:

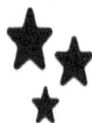

Verse of The Day: _____
_____
_____
_____

Prayer Requests:

Praise Reports:

Reflections: _____
_____
_____
_____
_____

Date:

Verse of The Day: _____
_____
_____
_____

Prayer Requests:

Praise Reports:

Reflections: _____
_____
_____
_____
_____

Date:

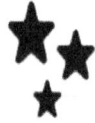

Verse of The Day: _____
_____
_____
_____

Prayer Requests:

Praise Reports:

Reflections: _____
_____
_____
_____
_____

Date:

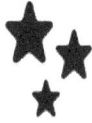

Verse of The Day: _____
_____
_____
_____

Prayer Requests:

Praise Reports:

Reflections: _____
_____
_____
_____
_____

Date:

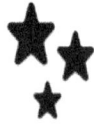

Verse of The Day: _____
_____
_____
_____

Prayer Requests:

Praise Reports:

Reflections: _____
_____
_____
_____
_____

Date:

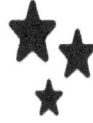

Verse of The Day: _____
_____
_____
_____

Prayer Requests:

Praise Reports:

Reflections: _____
_____
_____
_____
_____

Date: _____

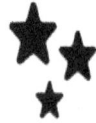

Verse of The Day: _____
_____
_____
_____

Prayer Requests:

Praise Reports:

Reflections: _____
_____
_____
_____
_____

Date:

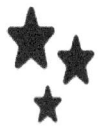

Verse of The Day: _____
_____
_____
_____

Prayer Requests:

Praise Reports:

Reflections: _____
_____
_____
_____
_____

Date:

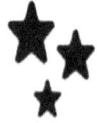

Verse of The Day: _____
_____
_____
_____

Prayer Requests:

Praise Reports:

Reflections: _____
_____
_____
_____
_____

Date:

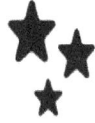

Verse of The Day: _____
_____
_____
_____

Prayer Requests:

Praise Reports:

Reflections: _____
_____
_____
_____
_____

Date:

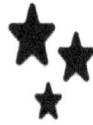

Verse of The Day: _____
_____
_____
_____

Prayer Requests:

Praise Reports:

Reflections: _____
_____
_____
_____
_____

Date:

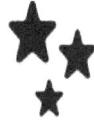

Verse of The Day: _____
_____
_____
_____

Prayer Requests:

Praise Reports:

Reflections: _____
_____
_____
_____
_____

Date:

Verse of The Day: _____
_____
_____
_____
_____

Prayer Requests:

Praise Reports:

Reflections: _____
_____
_____
_____
_____

Date:

Verse of The Day: _____
_____
_____
_____

Prayer Requests:

Praise Reports:

Reflections: _____
_____
_____
_____
_____

Date:

Verse of The Day: _____
_____
_____
_____

Prayer Requests:

Praise Reports:

Reflections: _____
_____
_____
_____
_____

Date:

Verse of The Day: _____
_____
_____
_____
_____

Prayer Requests:

Praise Reports:

Reflections: _____
_____
_____
_____
_____

Date:

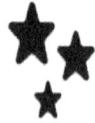

Verse of The Day: _____
_____
_____
_____

Prayer Requests:

Praise Reports:

Reflections: _____
_____
_____
_____
_____

Date:

Verse of The Day: _____
_____
_____
_____

Prayer Requests:

Praise Reports:

Reflections: _____
_____
_____
_____
_____

Date:

Verse of The Day:

_____
_____
_____
_____

Prayer Requests:

Praise Reports:

Reflections:

_____
_____
_____
_____

Date:

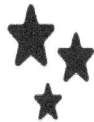

Verse of The Day: _____
_____
_____
_____

Prayer Requests:

Praise Reports:

Reflections: _____
_____
_____
_____
_____

Date:

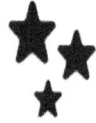

Verse of The Day: _____
_____
_____
_____

Prayer Requests:

Praise Reports:

Reflections: _____
_____
_____
_____
_____

Date:

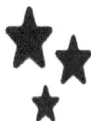

Verse of The Day: _____
_____
_____
_____

Prayer Requests:

Praise Reports:

Reflections: _____
_____
_____
_____
_____

Date:

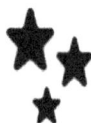

Verse of The Day: _____
_____
_____
_____

Prayer Requests:

Praise Reports:

Reflections: _____
_____
_____
_____
_____

Date:

Verse of The Day: _____
_____
_____
_____

Prayer Requests:

Praise Reports:

Reflections: _____
_____
_____
_____
_____

Date:

Verse of The Day: _____
_____
_____
_____

Prayer Requests:

Praise Reports:

Reflections: _____
_____
_____
_____
_____

Date:

Verse of The Day: _____
_____
_____
_____

Prayer Requests:

Praise Reports:

Reflections: _____
_____
_____
_____
_____

Date:

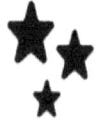

Verse of The Day: _____
_____
_____
_____

Prayer Requests:

Praise Reports:

Reflections: _____
_____
_____
_____
_____

Date:

Verse of The Day: _____
_____
_____
_____

Prayer Requests:

Praise Reports:

Reflections: _____
_____
_____
_____
_____

Date:

Verse of The Day: _____
_____
_____
_____

Prayer Requests:

Praise Reports:

Reflections: _____
_____
_____
_____
_____

Date:

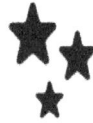

Verse of The Day: _____
_____
_____
_____

Prayer Requests:

Praise Reports:

Reflections: _____
_____
_____
_____
_____

Date:

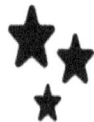

Verse of The Day: _____
_____
_____
_____

Prayer Requests:

Praise Reports:

Reflections: _____
_____
_____
_____
_____

Psalm 20:1

The Lord will hear
me, in
the day of trouble;
The name of the
God of Jacob will
defend me.

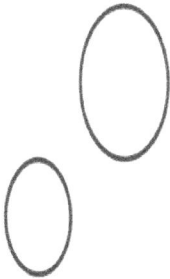

Date:

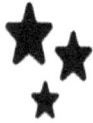

Verse of The Day: _____
_____
_____
_____

Prayer Requests:

Praise Reports:

Reflections: _____
_____
_____
_____
_____

Date:

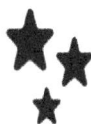

Verse of The Day: _____
_____
_____
_____

Prayer Requests:

Praise Reports:

Reflections: _____
_____
_____
_____
_____

Date:

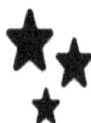

Verse of The Day: _____
_____
_____
_____

Prayer Requests:

Praise Reports:

Reflections: _____
_____
_____
_____
_____

Date:

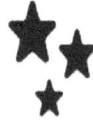

Verse of The Day: _____
_____
_____
_____

Prayer Requests:

Praise Reports:

Reflections: _____
_____
_____
_____
_____

Date:

Verse of The Day: _____
_____
_____
_____

Prayer Requests:

Praise Reports:

Reflections: _____
_____
_____
_____
_____

Date:

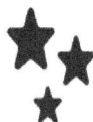

Verse of The Day: _____
_____
_____
_____

Prayer Requests:

Praise Reports:

Reflections: _____
_____
_____
_____
_____

Date:

Verse of The Day: _____
_____
_____
_____

Prayer Requests:

Praise Reports:

Reflections: _____
_____
_____
_____
_____

Date:

Verse of The Day: _____
_____
_____
_____

Prayer Requests:

Praise Reports:

Reflections: _____
_____
_____
_____
_____

Date:

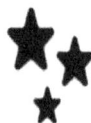

Verse of The Day: _____
_____
_____
_____

Prayer Requests:

Praise Reports:

Reflections:_____
_____
_____
_____
_____
_____

Date:

Verse of The Day: _____
_____
_____
_____

Prayer Requests:

Praise Reports:

Reflections: _____
_____
_____
_____
_____

Date:

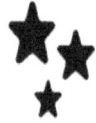

Verse of The Day: _____
_____
_____
_____

Prayer Requests:

Praise Reports:

Reflections: _____
_____
_____
_____
_____

Date:

Verse of The Day: _____
_____
_____
_____

Prayer Requests:

Praise Reports:

Reflections: _____
_____
_____
_____
_____

Date:

Verse of The Day: _____
_____
_____
_____

Prayer Requests:

Praise Reports:

Reflections: _____
_____
_____
_____
_____

Date:

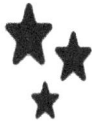

Verse of The Day: _____
_____
_____
_____

Prayer Requests:

Praise Reports:

Reflections: _____
_____
_____
_____
_____

Date:

Verse of The Day: _____
_____
_____
_____

Prayer Requests:

Praise Reports:

Reflections: _____
_____
_____
_____
_____

Date:

Verse of The Day: _____
_____
_____
_____

Prayer Requests:

Praise Reports:

Reflections: _____
_____
_____
_____
_____

Date:

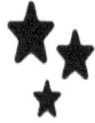

Verse of The Day: _____

_____

_____

_____

Prayer Requests:

Praise Reports:

Reflections: _____

_____

_____

_____

_____

Date:

Verse of The Day: _____
_____
_____
_____

Prayer Requests:

Praise Reports:

Reflections: _____
_____
_____
_____
_____

Date:

Verse of The Day: _____
_____
_____
_____

Prayer Requests:

Praise Reports:

Reflections: _____
_____
_____
_____
_____

Date:

Verse of The Day: _____
_____
_____
_____

Prayer Requests:

Praise Reports:

Reflections: _____
_____
_____
_____
_____

Date:

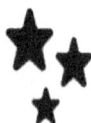

Verse of The Day: _____
_____
_____
_____

Prayer Requests:

Praise Reports:

Reflections: _____
_____
_____
_____
_____

Date:

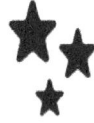

Verse of The Day: _____
_____
_____
_____

Prayer Requests:

Praise Reports:

Reflections: _____
_____
_____
_____
_____

Date:

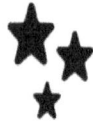

Verse of The Day: _____
_____
_____
_____

Prayer Requests:

Praise Reports:

Reflections: _____
_____
_____
_____
_____

Date:

Verse of The Day: _____
_____
_____
_____

Prayer Requests:

Praise Reports:

Reflections: _____
_____
_____
_____
_____

Date:

Verse of The Day: _____
_____
_____
_____

Prayer Requests:

Praise Reports:

Reflections: _____
_____
_____
_____
_____

Date:

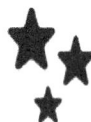

Verse of The Day: _____

_____

_____

_____

Prayer Requests:

Praise Reports:

Reflections: _____

_____

_____

_____

_____

Date: _____

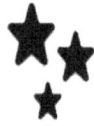

Verse of The Day: _____
_____
_____
_____

Prayer Requests:

Praise Reports:

Reflections: _____
_____
_____
_____
_____

Date:

Verse of The Day:

Prayer Requests:

Praise Reports:

Reflections:

Date:

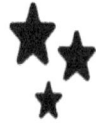

Verse of The Day: _____
_____
_____
_____

Prayer Requests:

Praise Reports:

Reflections: _____
_____
_____
_____
_____

Date:

Verse of The Day: _____
_____
_____
_____

Prayer Requests:

Praise Reports:

Reflections: _____
_____
_____
_____
_____

Date:

Verse of The Day: _____
_____
_____
_____

Prayer Requests:

Praise Reports:

Reflections: _____
_____
_____
_____
_____

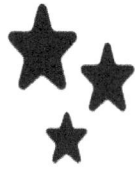

Psalm 91:15

I will call upon the
Lord, and he will
answer me;
He will be with me in
trouble; He will
deliver me
and honor me.

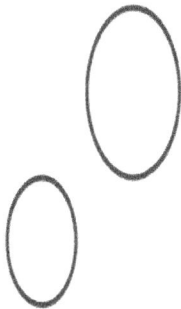

Ideas For Selfcare ★★★

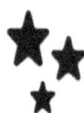

- ✓ Take a mental health day, and do not feel an ounce of guilt about it
- ✓ Burn a candle or diffuse some oils that have scents that bring you joy
- ✓ Walk around the grocery store without a list; Buy some stuff just for fun
- ✓ Go to the library or bookstore; Sit in a comfy chair and read
- ✓ Sing at the top of your lungs, in the car, with the windows down
- ✓ Do something crafty: coloring, knitting, sewing…..
- ✓ Take a bubble bath with candles and calming music
- ✓ Sit in a coffee shop and sip on a luxurious drink
- ✓ Sit on the front porch; Just sit and do nothing
- ✓ Sit in the grass and watch the clouds float by
- ✓ Pick or buy a bouquet of fresh flowers
- ✓ Go for a drive - no destination required
- ✓ Have a dance party to your favorite music
- ✓ Wrap yourself in a soft, warm blanket
- ✓ Give yourself a pedicure or a manicure
- ✓ Read a book or magazine for an hour
- ✓ Take a leisurely walk without a goal
- ✓ Put on a homemade face mask
- ✓ Watch funny YouTube videos
- ✓ Try out a new hobby
- ✓ Look at the stars
- ✓ Sit in the sun
- ✓ Meditate
- ✓ Take a nap
- ✓ Write in your Journal

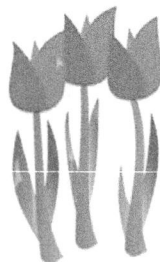

Inspiration

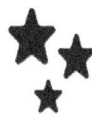

As a Christian woman there are so many wonderful moments that I have experienced with The Lord that have caused me to rejoice and to be filled with hope for the future, no matter what I am going through. I often recount these moments to others; including my children, family members, friends and church family. I realized it would have been so much easier to recount some of these experiences to uplift the people that I am talking to by reading from my journals instead of trying to remember all the details from memory.

I created this journal, to help my fellow believers around the world to be embolden to document and share their encounters with God and proudly capture his greatness. This will help you to pass on great inspirational stories and spiritual traditions to the next generation and to encourage you to bring others into the presence of God.

My hope is that this journal will encourage you to record your thoughts and beliefs, to record those inspirational moments that have helped to bring you closer to the Lord and also to develop within you an attitude of gratitude and praise for all the wonderful miracles that God has worked in your life.

Deuteronomy 7:9 - Know therefore that the LORD your God is God; he is the faithful God, keeping his covenant of love to a thousand generations of those who love him and keep his commandments.

-A.R. Francis

My Reflections:

_____
_____
_____
_____
_____
_____
_____
_____
_____
_____
_____
_____
_____
_____
_____
_____
_____
_____
_____
_____
_____
_____
_____

My Reflections:

_____
_____
_____
_____
_____
_____
_____
_____
_____
_____
_____
_____
_____
_____
_____
_____
_____
_____
_____
_____
_____
_____

My Reflections:

_____
_____
_____
_____
_____
_____
_____
_____
_____
_____
_____
_____
_____
_____
_____
_____
_____
_____
_____
_____
_____

Made in the USA
Las Vegas, NV
07 April 2021